ISBN: 978-0-6459403-4-3

Published by How2Books
Under licence from MSI Ltd, Australia
Company Registration No: 96963518255
NSW, Australia

See our website: www.how2books.com.au
Or contact by email: admin@booksforreadingonline.com
Covers and Copyright owned by MSI, Australia

MSI acknowledges the author and images, text and photographs used in this book.

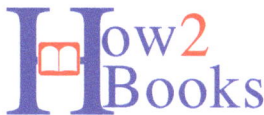

How2
Books

PLEASE WORK WITH YOUR BOOK:
'Grandma's Personal Trainer'
While you become familiar with your exercises and getting to know how your body works as you exercise.

SETTING GOALS – MODULE ONE

ARM EXERCISES

Arm movements and rotations

Keeping your eye on your health and wellbeing can only be a great goal, so let's start right now.

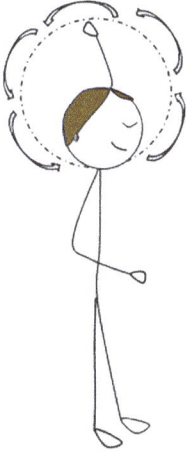

With setting your goal to start exercising you need a day. I suggest your write down your goals the night or day before and then you are prepared to work on exercises the following day. By adding the date of the exercise, it will help you to monitor your progress.

YOUR GOAL – ARM ROTATIONS

....

....

....

....

....

....

....

....

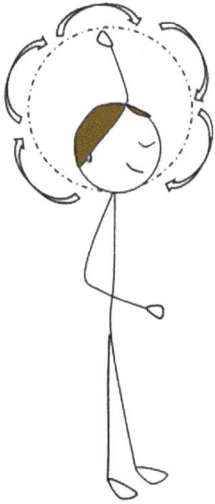

ARM AND HAND UPWARD STRETCHING

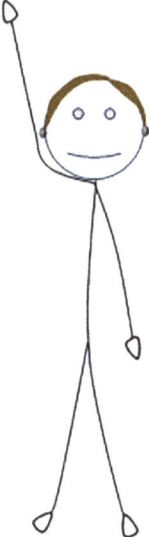

....

....

....

....

....

....

....

....

....

....

....

....

....

....

....

....

....

....

....

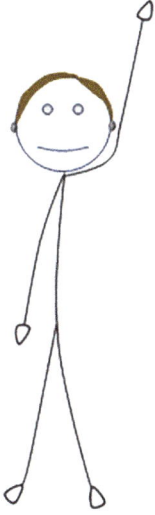

'STRETCH', 'STRETCH', 'STRETCH'

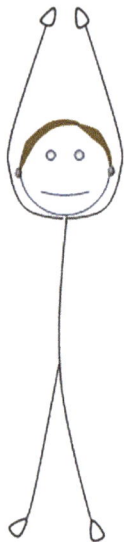

....
....
....
....
....
....
....
....
....
....
....
....
....
....
....
....
....
....
....

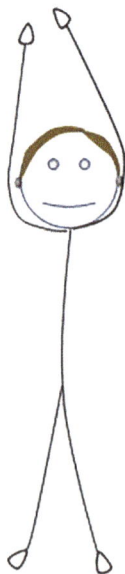
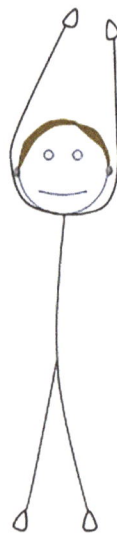

ROLLING YOUR SHOULDERS

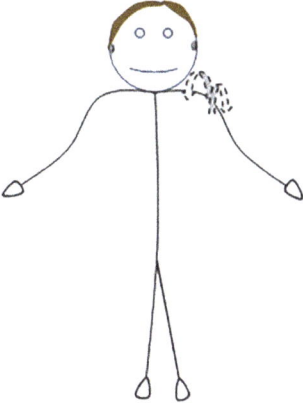

....
....
....
....
....
....
....
....
....
....
....

....
....
....
....
....
....
....
....

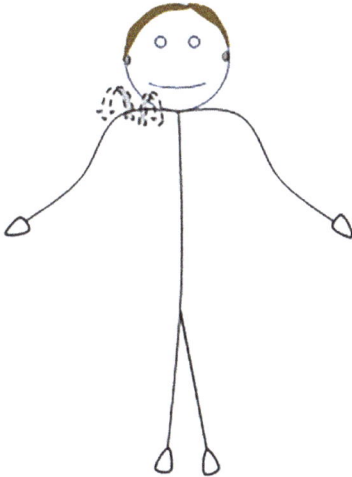

BOTH ARM ROTATIONS

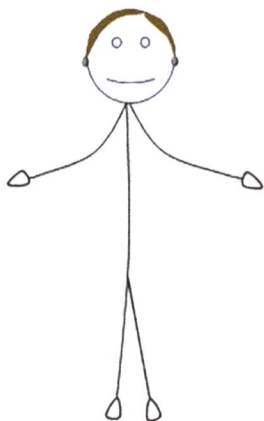

1)

....
....
....
....
....
....
....

2)

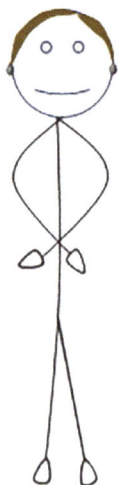

....
....
....
....
....
....
....
....
....

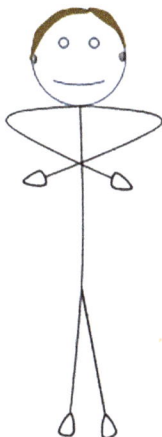

3)

....
....
....
....
....
....
....
....

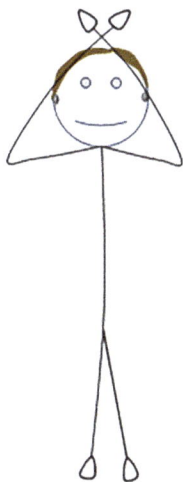

4)

....
....
....
....
....
....
....
....
....

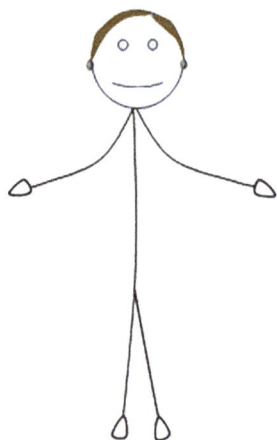

5)

....
....
....
....
....
....
....
....
....
....
....
....
....
....
....
....
....
....
....

SETTING GOALS - MODULE TWO
BREATHING – MOVING YOUR LEGS, ANKLES AND FEET

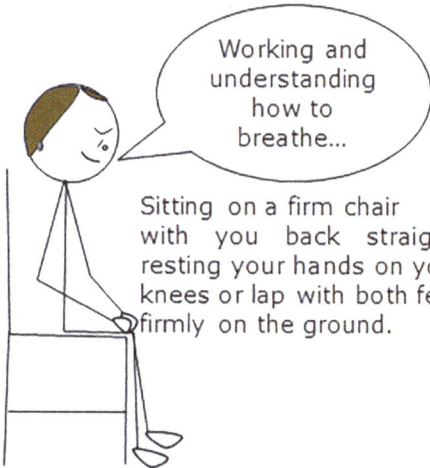

Working and understanding how to breathe...

Sitting on a firm chair with you back straight, resting your hands on your knees or lap with both feet firmly on the ground.

....

....

....

....

....

....

....

....

....

Lift your head high and feel proud of who you are.

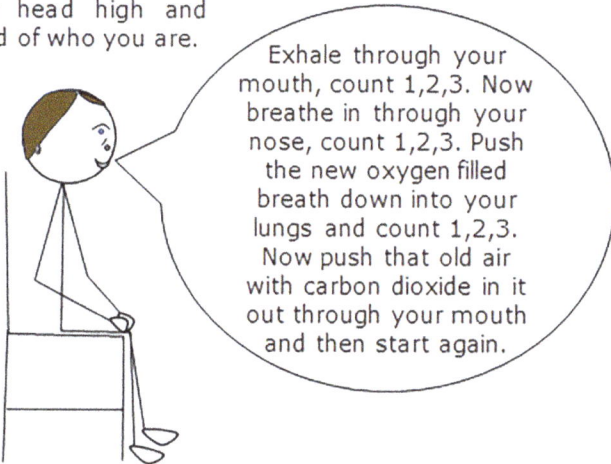

Exhale through your mouth, count 1,2,3. Now breathe in through your nose, count 1,2,3. Push the new oxygen filled breath down into your lungs and count 1,2,3. Now push that old air with carbon dioxide in it out through your mouth and then start again.

KEEPING A RECORD OF YOUR BREATHING REGIME

....

....

....

....

....

....

....

....

....

....

....

....

....

....

....

....

....

....

SIDE TO SIDE HEAD MOVEMENTS

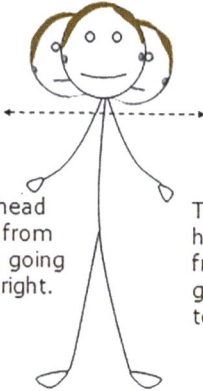

Five gentle head movements from side to side, going from left to right.

Then five gentle head movements from side to side, going from right to left.

FORWARD AND BACK HEAD MOVEMENTS

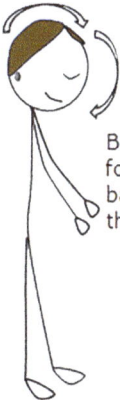

Bring your head forward, then back, forward, then back...

BACK AND FORWARD HEAD MOVEMENTS

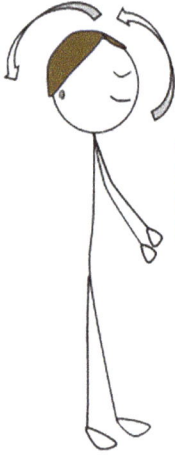

Bring your head back, then forward, then back...

....
....
....
....
....
....
....
....
....
....
....

WRIST MOVEMENTS AND ROTATIONS

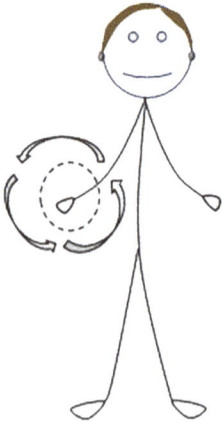

....
....
....
....
....
....
....

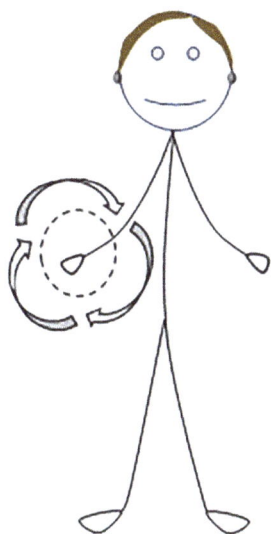

....

....

....

....

....

....

....

....

....

....

....

....

....

....

....

....

....

....

....

SETTING GOALS – MODULE THREE
YOUR BRAIN, THE FOOD YOU EAT...! EXERCISING YOUR LEGS, ANKLES AND FEET

Standing can help to
re-align your body weight.

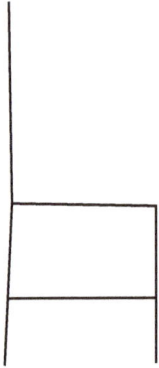

....

....

....

....

....

....

....

....

....

STANDING ON ONE LEG, COUNT TO TEN

....

....

....

....

....

....

....

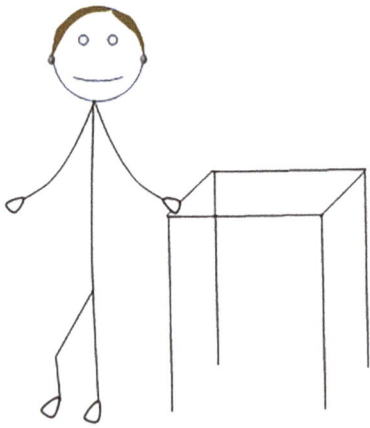

CHANGE TO YOUR OTHER LEG AND COUNT TO TEN

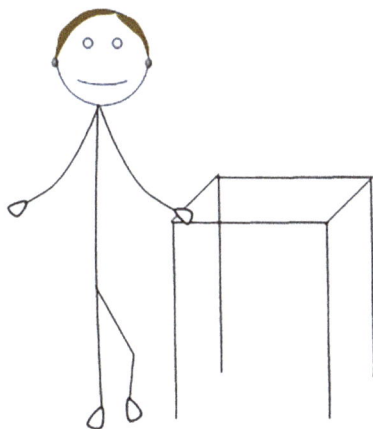

....

....

....

....

....

....

....

....

ROTATING YOUR FOOT – LEFT THEN RIGHT

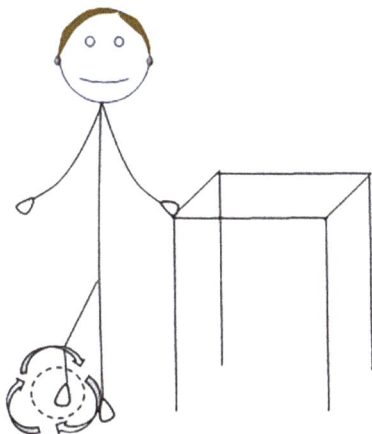

....

....

....

....

....

....

....

....

....

....

15

AND NOW THE OTHER ANKLE

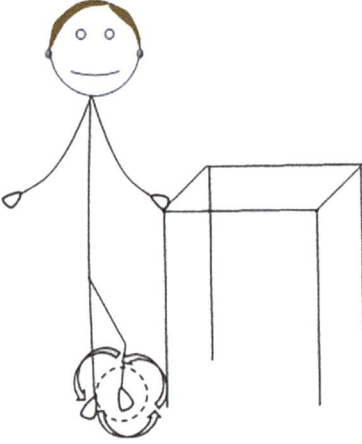

....

....

....

....

....

....

....

....

....

....

....

....

....

....

....

....

....

....

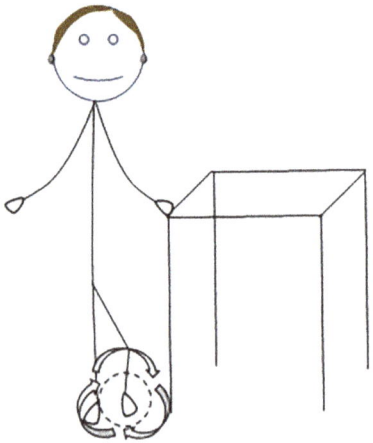

MOVING YOUR TOES IN THE DIRECTION OF YOUR KNEE

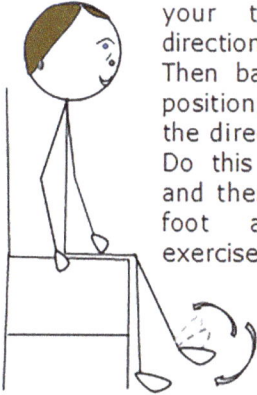

Sitting back on the chair and while your ankles and feet are limbered up, bring your toes up in the direction of the knee.
Then back to the original position, then back up into the direction of your knee. Do this five to ten times and then go to your other foot and repeat the exercise.

....

....

....

....

....

....

....

....

....

....

....

....

....

....

....

....

....

....

....

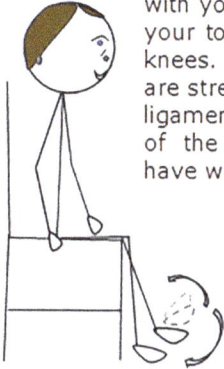

Now repeat the exercise with your other foot. Bring your toes up to meet your knees. By doing this you are stretching the tendons, ligaments and other areas of the foot that need to have workouts...!

STENGTHENING YOUR ANKLES AND LEGS

Other ways of strengthening your feet and ankle muscles can be done while sitting on a chair, securing a large elastic band to a secure post, such as a bed post and pulling your leg and foot backwards and forwards.

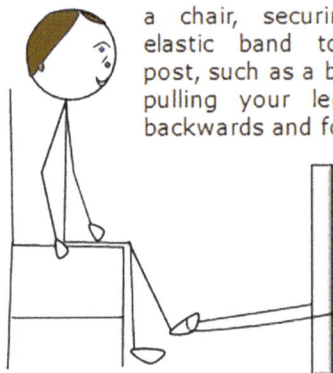

....

....

....

....

....

....

....

....

....

....

STRENGTHENING YOUR ANKLES AND FEET

Exercising the bottom of your foot is equally as important as exercising other areas of your feet and body.

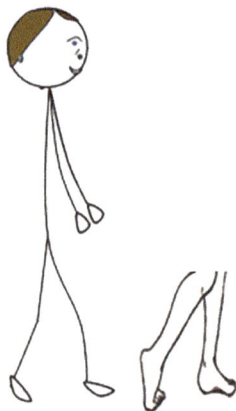

....

....

....

....

....

....
....
....
....
....
....
....
....
....

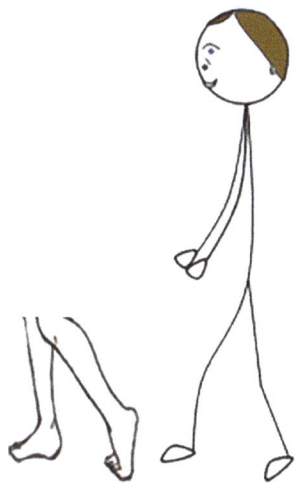

PAYING MORE ATTENTION TO YOUR LEGS – SIDEWAYS MOVEMENTS – SWEEPING YOUR LEG OUT AND BACK

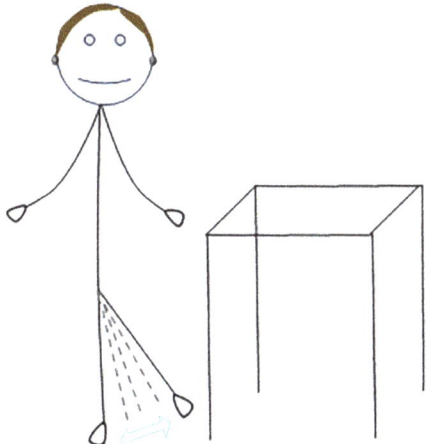

....
....
....
....
....
....
....

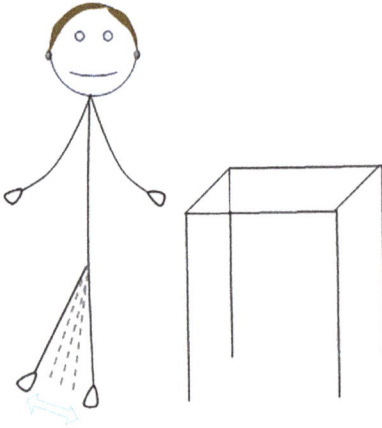

....
....
....
....
....
....
....
....
....

USING YOUR LEGS TO THEIR MAXIMUM ADVANTAGE – STAND UP – SIT DOWN

....
....
....
....
....
....
....
....

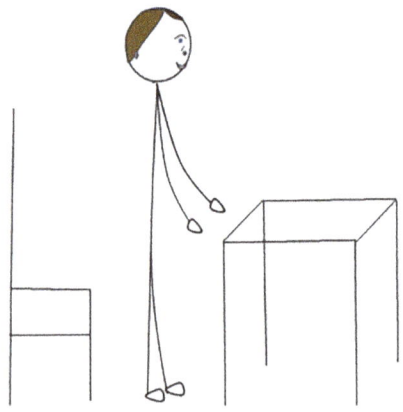

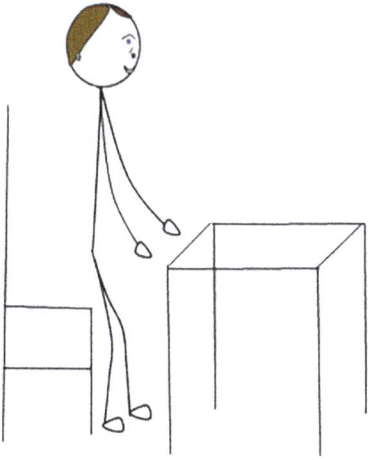

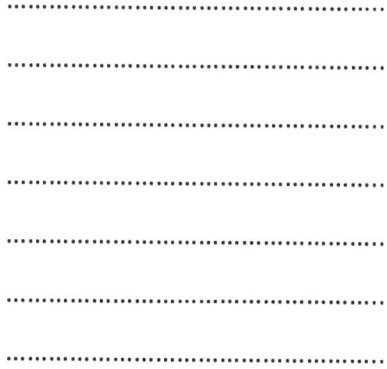

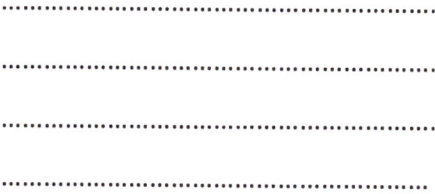

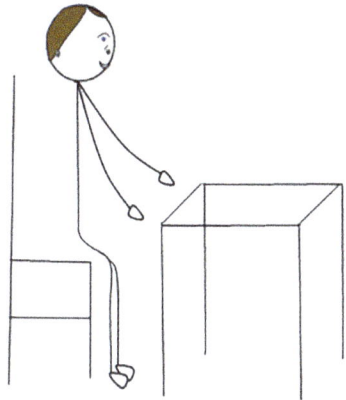

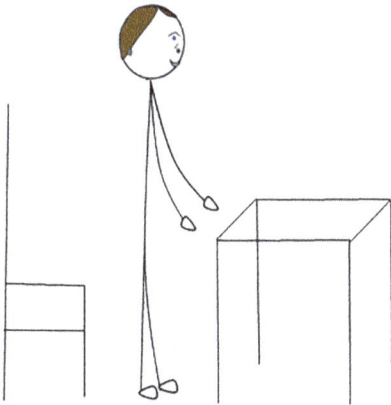

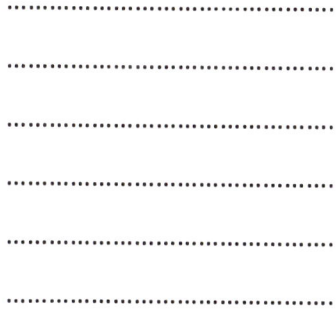

SETTING GOALS - MODULE FOUR
THE MOLECULES IN YOUR FOOD AND DRINK – KNEE LIFTS AND MORE LEG EXERCISES

RAISING YOUR KNEES

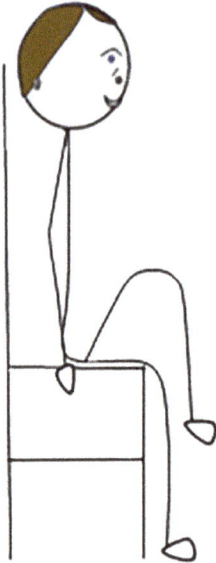

....

....

....

....

....

....

....

....

....

....

....

....

....

....

....

....

TUMMY IN, BACKSIDE OUT, LEGS SLIGHTLY APART

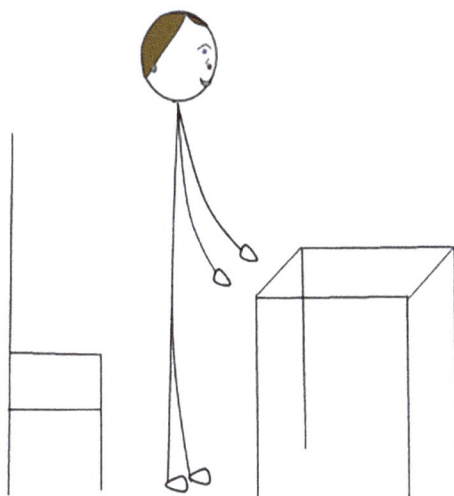

....
....
....
....
....
....
....
....
....
....

....
....
....
....
....
....
....
....

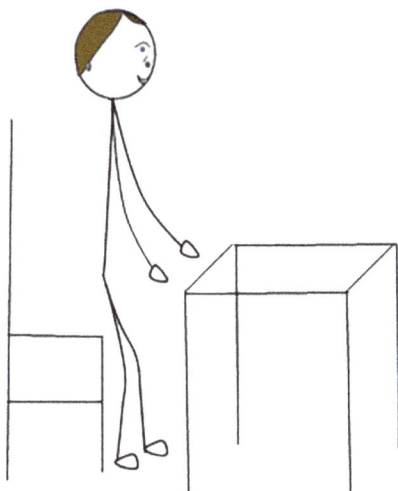

LEARNING TO SQUAT AGAIN...! TO BEGIN THE SQUAT - STAND UP STRAIGHT

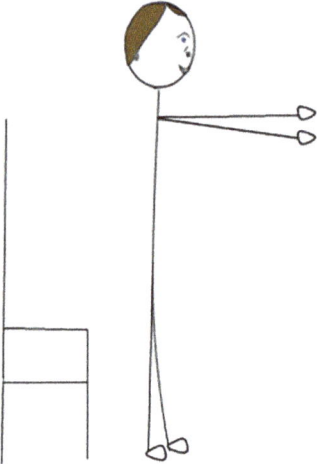

....
....
....
....
....
....
....
....
....

....

....
....
....
....
....
....
....
....

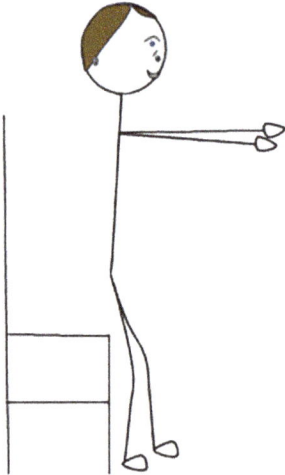

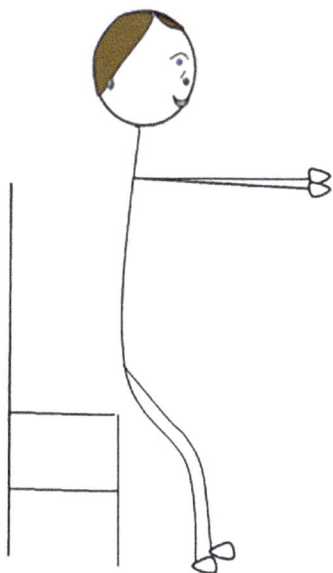

....
....
....
....
....
....
....
....
....
....

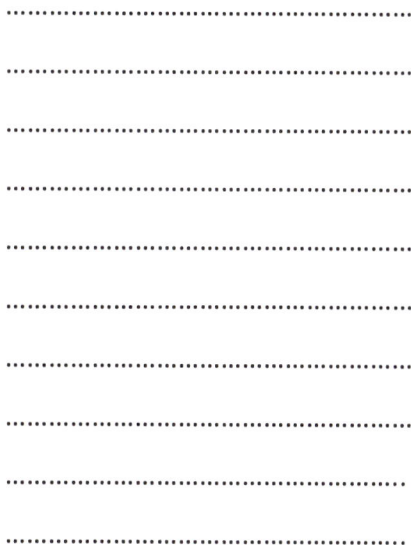

....
....
....
....
....
....
....
....
....
....

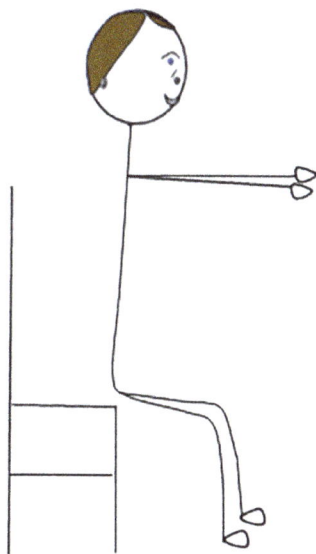

WALL SQUATS

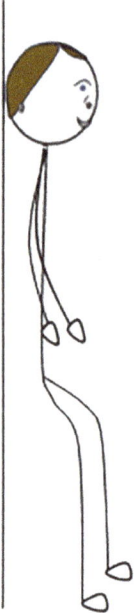

....
....
....
....
....
....
....
....
....
....
....

BENDING YOUR KNEES AND
LOWERING YOUR BODY – WALL
SQUATS

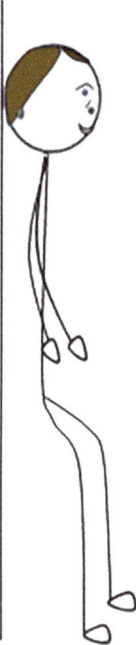

....
....
....
....
....
....

SETTING GOALS – MODULE FIVE
KNOWING ABOUT GELATINE AND MARROWBONE - LEG RAISING AND GLUTE BRIDGING, STRENGTHENING YOUR LOWER BODY EXERCISES

LEG RAISING EXERCISE – USING YOUR QUADS

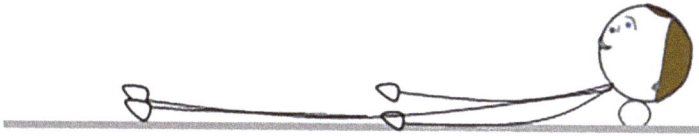

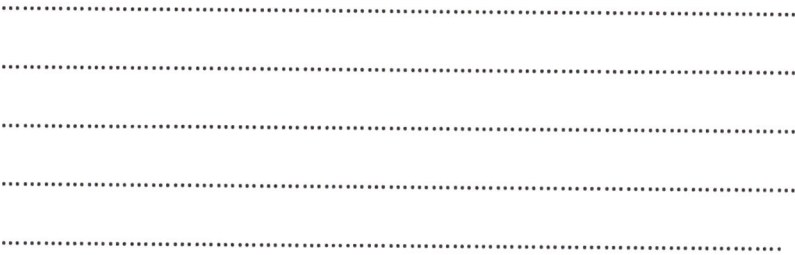

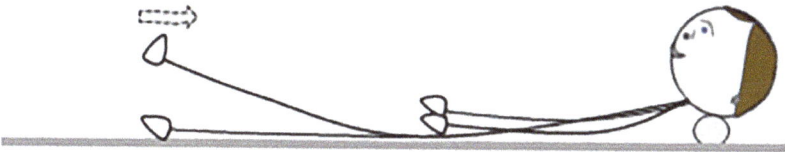

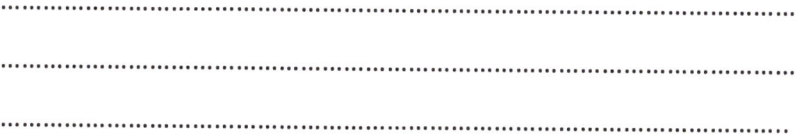

....
....
....
....
....

....
....
....

GLUTE BRIDGING AND STRENGTHENING YOUR LOWER BODY

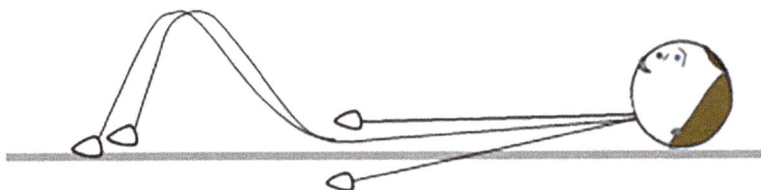

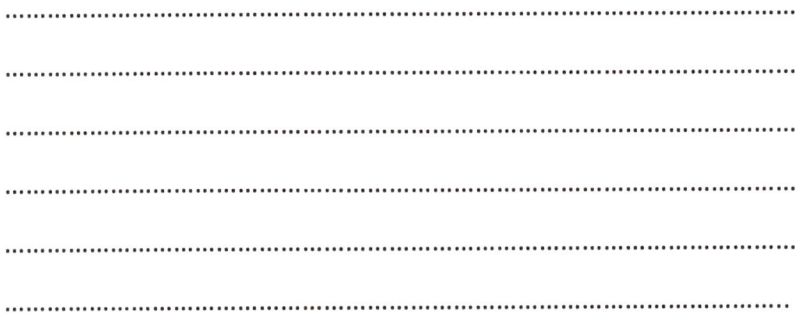

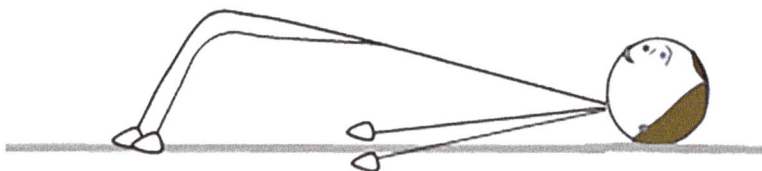

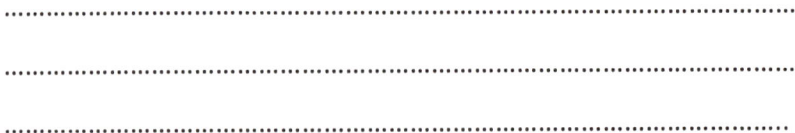

....

....

....

....

....

....

....

....

....

www.ingramcontent.com/pod-product-compliance
Lightning Source LLC
Chambersburg PA
CBHW041302040426

42334CB00028BA/3128